Mediterranean Seafood for Beginners

Quick and Easy Mediterranean Recipes to Boost Your Health and Improve Your Skills

Raymond Morton

Table of contents

Walnuts Salmon..6

Salmon with Brussels Sprouts...............................8

Salmon with Ginger...10

Cilantro Trout and Olives.....................................12

Salmon with Rice...14

Chives and Chili Salmon..16

Coconut and Parsley Salmon................................18

Smoked Trout and Avocado Bowls......................20

Shrimp, Onion and Spinach Salad......................22

Saffron Cloves Shrimp..24

Salmon and Rosemary Mix...................................26

Shrimp and Coriander Tomatoes........................28

Orange Shrimp...30

Trout with Scallions and Green Beans...............32

Cinnamon Cod...34

Salmon and Cantaloupe Salad.............................36

Cayenne Sea Bass and Olives...............................38

Salmon with Leeks...40

Curry and Coconut Halibut....................................42

Salmon and Rosemary Sweet Potatoes..............44

Salmon with Herbs...46

Shrimp and Pinto Beans...48

Shrimp with Baby Spinach.....................................50

Cod and Peppers...52

Cod with Avocado and Peppers Pan....................54

Shrimp and Zucchinis..56

Lemon Rosemary Scallops..58

Crab and Kale Salad..60

Salmon with Paprika Tomatoes..62

Shrimp and Mango Salad..64

Creamy Cod...66

Trout and Walnuts Cilantro Sauce..................................68

Cilantro Tilapia..70

Salmon and Green Chilies Mix..72

Salmon and Green Chilies Mix..74

Shrimp and Turmeric Cauliflower Mix...........................76

Tuna with Broccoli..78

Flounder with Mushrooms...80

Spicy Shrimp with Rice...82

Dill Sea Bass...84

Trout with Coconut Tomato Sauce..................................86

Salmon and Cilantro Roasted Peppers..........................88

Lemon and Garlic Shrimp and Beets..............................90

Parsley and Lime Shrimp...92

Cumin Shrimp and Almonds..95

Tilapia and Red Beans...97

Shrimp with Corn and Olives...99

Citrus Scallops..101

Shrimp with Leeks and Carrots.....................................103

Cod and Barley..105

Shrimp and Balsamic Sweet Peppers..........................107

Cumin Snapper Mix..109

Walnuts Salmon

Prep time: 10 minutes I **Cooking time:** 20 minutes I
Servings: 4

Ingredients:

- 4 salmon fillets, boneless
- 2 tablespoons olive oil
- 2 tablespoons walnuts, chopped
- 1 tablespoon parsley, chopped
- 2 tablespoons vegetable stock
- 1 teaspoon rosemary, dried
- Salt and black pepper to the taste

Directions:

1. In a roasting pan, combine the salmon with the oil, the walnuts and the other ingredients, toss gently and cook at 380 degrees F for 20 minutes.
2. Divide the mix between plates and serve with a side salad.

Nutrition info per serving: calories 323, fat 20.9, fiber 0.4, carbs 1.1, protein 35.5

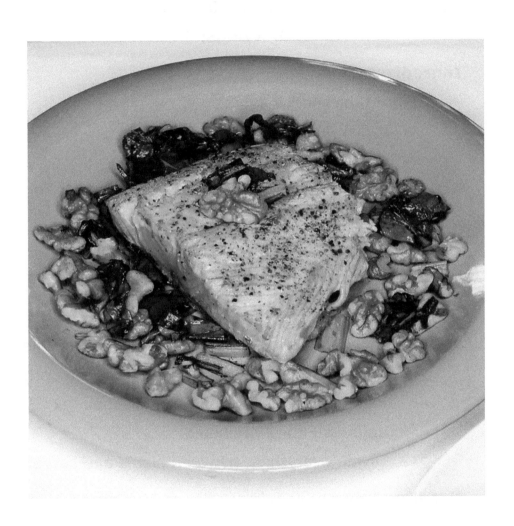

Salmon with Brussels Sprouts

Prep time: 5 minutes I **Cooking time:** 20 minutes I
Servings: 4

Ingredients:

- 2 tablespoons avocado oil
- 1 cup brussels sprouts
- 4 salmon fillets, skinless
- 1 teaspoon chili powder
- 1 teaspoon cumin, ground
- 1 tablespoon chives, chopped
- A pinch of sea salt and black pepper

Directions:

1. In a baking dish, combine the salmon fillets with the oil, the broccoli and the other ingredients, toss gently and cook at 380 degrees F for 20 minutes.
2. Divide everything between plates and serve.

Nutrition info per serving: calories 257, fat 12.2, fiber 1.2, carbs 2.5, protein 35.5

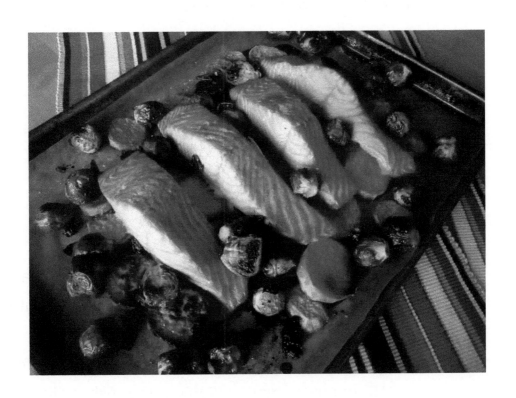

Salmon with Ginger

Prep time: 10 minutes I **Cooking time:** 20 minutes I **Servings:** 4

Ingredients:

- 4 salmon fillets, boneless
- 4 scallions, chopped
- 2 tablespoons avocado oil
- 2 garlic cloves, minced
- 1 tablespoon ginger, grated
- 1 teaspoon turmeric powder
- 1 teaspoon rosemary, dried
- 1 tablespoon parsley, chopped

Directions:

1. Heat up a pan with the oil over medium heat, add the scallions, garlic and ginger and sauté for 5 minutes.
2. Add the fish and the other ingredients, cook for 15 minutes more, flipping the fish halfway, divide between plates and serve.

Nutrition info per serving: calories 260, fat 12.1, fiber 1.2, carbs 3.6, protein 35.2

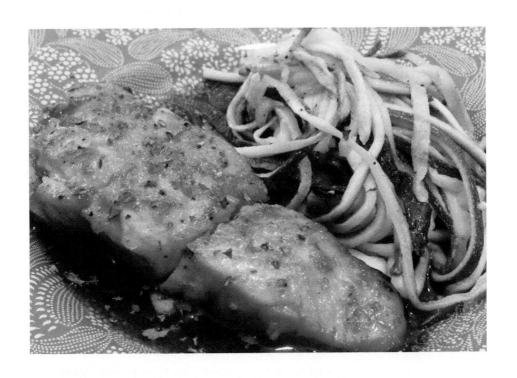

Cilantro Trout and Olives

Prep time: 10 minutes I **Cooking time:** 30 minutes I
Servings: 4

Ingredients:

- 4 trout fillets, boneless
- 1 cup green olives, pitted
- 2 tablespoons olive oil
- ½ teaspoon smoked paprika
- ½ teaspoon cumin, ground
- Salt and black pepper to the taste
- ¼ cup vegetable stock
- 2 tablespoons cilantro, chopped

Directions:

1. In a roasting pan, combine the trout fillets with the olives, the oil and the other ingredients, toss gently and cook at 380 degrees F for 30 minutes.
2. Divide the mix between plates and serve.

Nutrition info per serving: calories 191, fat 13.6, fiber 0.4, carbs 1.4, protein 16.7

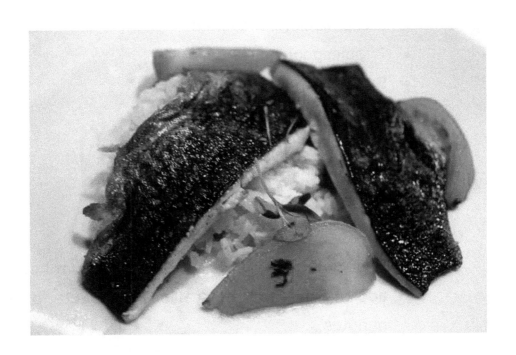

Salmon with Rice

Prep time: 5 minutes I **Cooking time:** 20 minutes I
Servings: 4

Ingredients:

- 4 salmon fillets, boneless and cubed
- ½ cup snow peas, blanched
- 1 cup black rice, cooked
- 2 tablespoons olive oil
- Salt and pepper to the taste
- 4 scallions, chopped
- 1 red chili, chopped
- Juice of 1 lime
- 1 tablespoon chives, chopped

Directions:

1. Heat up a pan with the oil over medium heat, add the chili and the scallions and sauté for 5 minutes.
2. Add the fish and cook it for 5 minutes more.
3. Add the peas, rice and the remaining ingredients, toss, cook over medium heat for 10 more minutes, divide into bowls and serve.

Nutrition info per serving: calories 354, fat 18.8, fiber 2, carbs 10.5, protein 37.5

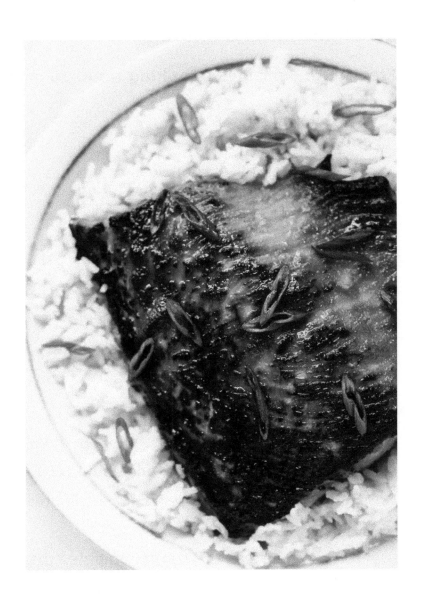

Chives and Chili Salmon

Prep time: 5 minutes I **Cooking time:** 15 minutes I
Servings: 4

Ingredients:

- 4 salmon fillets, boneless
- 1 teaspoon chili powder
- 1 teaspoon hot paprika
- 2 tablespoons olive oil
- 2 spring onions, chopped
- A pinch of salt and black pepper
- ¼ cup fresh chives, chopped
- 1 tablespoon lemon juice

Directions:

1. Heat up a pan with the oil over medium heat, add the spring onions and sauté for 2 minutes.
2. Add the fish and cook it for 5 minutes on each side.
3. Add the rest of the ingredients, toss gently, cook for 3 minutes more, divide everything between plates and serve.

Nutrition info per serving: calories 272, fat 4, fiber 2, carbs 12, protein 7

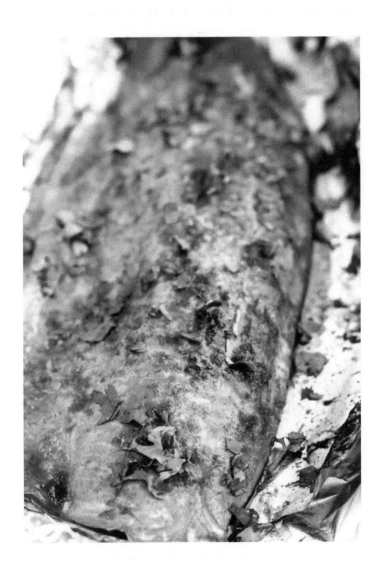

Coconut and Parsley Salmon

Prep time: 5 minutes I **Cooking time:** 14 minutes I
Servings: 4

Ingredients:

- 1 cup coconut cream
- 4 salmon fillets, boneless
- 2 tablespoons avocado oil
- 4 scallions, chopped
- 1 tablespoon parsley, chopped
- 1 tablespoon lemon juice
- A pinch of salt and black pepper

Directions:

1. Heat up a pan with the oil over medium-high heat, add the scallions and sauté for 4 minutes.
2. Add the fish and cook it for 3 minutes on each side.
3. Add the rest of the ingredients, toss gently, cook for 4 minutes more, divide between plates and serve.

Nutrition info per serving: calories 215, fat 3, fiber 2, carbs 8, protein 6

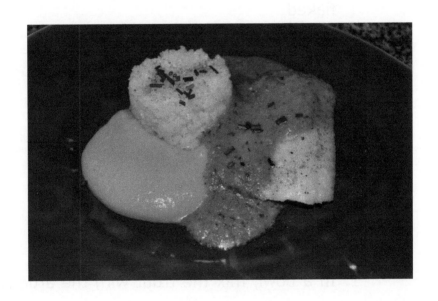

Smoked Trout and Avocado Bowls

Prep time: 10 minutes I **Cooking time:** 0 minutes I **Servings:** 4

Ingredients:

- 1 pound smoked trout, boneless, skinless and flaked
- 1 cup baby arugula
- 2 tablespoons lemon juice
- 2 tomatoes, cubed
- 1 avocado, peeled, pitted and cubed
- 1 tablespoon chives, minced
- 1 tablespoon olive oil
- A pinch of salt and black pepper

Directions:

1. In a bowl, mix the trout with the arugula and the other ingredients, toss and serve.

Nutrition info per serving: calories 200, fat 7, fiber 3, carbs 12, protein 6

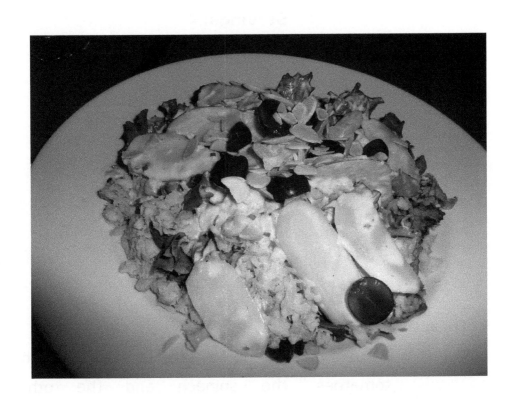

21

Shrimp, Onion and Spinach Salad

Prep time: 5 minutes I **Cooking time:** 0 minutes I
Servings: 4

Ingredients:

- 3 tablespoons balsamic vinegar
- 2 tablespoons olive oil
- 2 garlic cloves, minced
- A pinch of salt and black pepper
- 1 pound shrimp, cooked, peeled and deveined
- ½ pound cherry tomatoes, halved
- ½ red onion, sliced
- 1 cup baby spinach

Directions:

1. In a bowl, combine the shrimp with the tomatoes, the spinach and the other ingredients, toss and serve.

Nutrition info per serving: calories 212, fat 7.3, fiber 3, carbs 6, protein 7

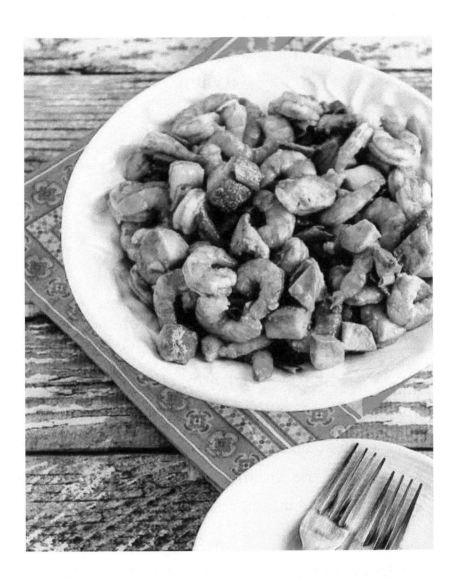

Saffron Cloves Shrimp

Prep time: 5 minutes I **Cooking time:** 8 minutes I
Servings: 4

Ingredients:

- 1 pound shrimp, peeled and deveined
- 1 tablespoon lemon juice
- ½ teaspoon sweet paprika
- 2 tablespoons olive oil
- 1 teaspoon saffron powder
- 1 teaspoon coriander, ground
- 1 teaspoon orange zest, grated
- ½ teaspoon cloves, ground
- 1 tablespoon cilantro, chopped

Directions:

1. Heat up a pan with the oil over medium heat,
   add the shrimp, lemon juice, saffron and the
   other ingredients, toss, cook for 8 minutes,
   divide the mix intro bowls and serve.

Nutrition info per serving: calories 230, fat 6.2, fiber
5, carbs 8, protein 4

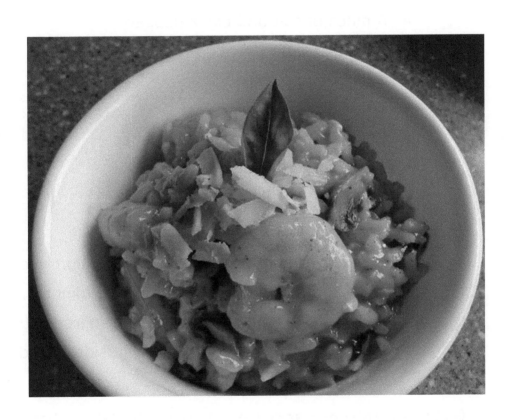

Salmon and Rosemary Mix

Prep time: 5 minutes I **Cooking time:** 14 minutes I
Servings: 4

Ingredients:

- 4 salmon fillets, boneless
- A pinch of salt and black pepper
- Juice of 1 lime
- 1 fennel bulb, sliced
- 2 tablespoons olive oil
- ½ teaspoon fennel seeds, crushed
- 1 teaspoon rosemary, dried
- 1 tablespoon cilantro, chopped

Directions:

1. Heat up a pan with the oil over medium-high heat, add the fennel and sauté for 2 minutes.
2. Add the fish and the rest of the ingredients, cook it for 6 minutes on each side, divide between plates and serve.

Nutrition info per serving: calories 200, fat 2, fiber 4, carbs 10, protein 8

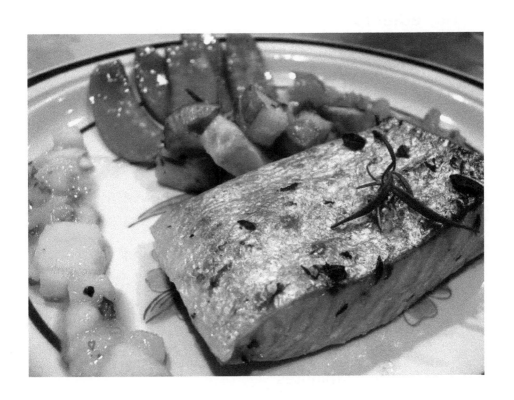

Shrimp and Coriander Tomatoes

Prep time: 5 minutes I **Cooking time:** 8 minutes I
Servings: 4

Ingredients:

- 1 pound shrimp, peeled and deveined
- 2 tablespoons olive oil
- 1 cup tomatoes, cubed
- 1 tablespoon lime juice
- 3 garlic cloves, minced
- A pinch of salt and black pepper
- ¼ cup pine nuts, toasted
- 2 tablespoons coriander, ground

Directions:

1. Heat up a pan with the oil over medium-high heat, add the garlic and the pine nuts and cook for 2 minutes.
2. Add the shrimp and the other ingredients, toss, cook over medium heat for 6 minutes, divide into bowls and serve.

Nutrition info per serving: calories 211, fat 10, fiber 4, carbs 5, protein 14

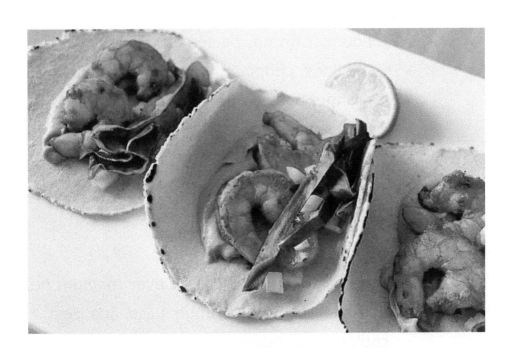

Orange Shrimp

Prep time: 5 minutes I **Cooking time:** 8 minutes I
Servings: 4

Ingredients:

- 2 pounds shrimp, peeled and deveined
- 2 scallions, chopped
- 1 orange, peeled and cut into segments
- 2 tablespoons olive oil
- ½ cup orange juice
- 1 tablespoon orange zest, grated
- 2 tablespoons chives, chopped

Directions:

1. Heat up a pan with the oil over medium heat,
   add the scallions, orange juice and zest and
   cook for 2 minutes.
2. Add the shrimp and the remaining ingredients,
   toss, cook for 6 minutes more, divide into bowls
   and serve.

Nutrition info per serving: calories 210, fat 6, fiber 4,
carbs 8, protein 14

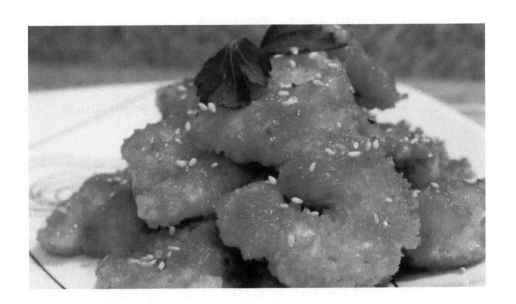

Trout with Scallions and Green Beans

Prep time: 5 minutes I **Cooking time:** 12 minutes I
Servings: 4

Ingredients:

- 4 trout fillets, boneless
- 2 tablespoons olive oil
- 4 scallions, chopped
- 1 cup green beans, trimmed and halved
- 1 tablespoon lemon juice
- 2 tablespoons cilantro, chopped

Directions:

1. Heat up a pan with the oil over medium-high heat, add the scallions and sauté for 2 minutes.
2. Add the fish and the other ingredients, cook for 5 minutes on each side, divide everything between plates and serve.

Nutrition info per serving: calories 209, fat 9, fiber 6, carbs 8, protein 14

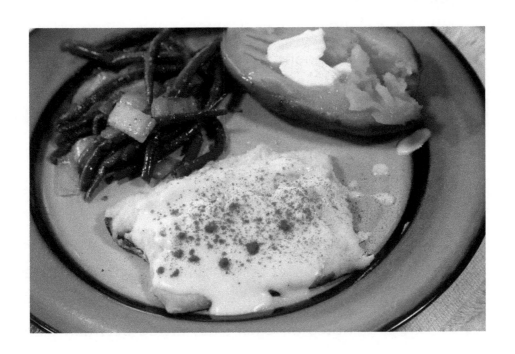

Cinnamon Cod

Prep time: 5 minutes I **Cooking time:** 12 minutes I **Servings:** 4

Ingredients:

- 4 cod fillets, boneless
- 2 tablespoons olive oil
- 1 tablespoon cinnamon powder
- ½ cup spring onions, chopped
- A pinch of salt and black pepper
- Juice of 1 lime

Directions:

1. Heat up a pan with the oil over medium heat, add the spring onions and sauté for 2 minutes.
2. Add the fish and the other ingredients, cook for 5 minutes on each side, divide between plates and serve.

Nutrition info per serving: calories 210, fat 12, fiber 4, carbs 7, protein 14

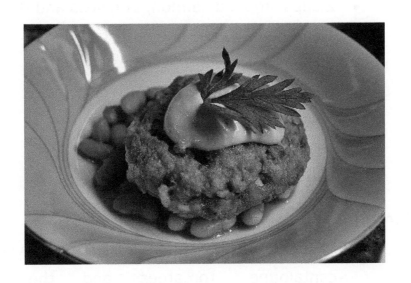

Salmon and Cantaloupe Salad

Prep time: 5 minutes I **Cooking time:** 0 minutes I
Servings: 4

Ingredients:

- 2 cups smoked salmon, boneless and flaked
- 1 cup cantaloupe, peeled and cubed
- 2 tomatoes, cubed
- 1 cucumber, sliced
- 2 tablespoons olive oil
- 1 tablespoon lime juice
- Salt and black pepper to the taste

Directions:

1. In a salad bowl, combine the salmon with the cantaloupe, tomatoes and the other ingredients, toss and serve.

Nutrition info per serving: calories 169, fat 2, fiber 2, carbs 12, protein 17

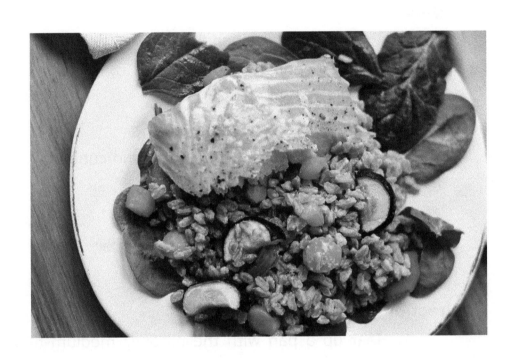

Cayenne Sea Bass and Olives

Prep time: 5 minutes I **Cooking time:** 14 minutes I
Servings: 4

Ingredients:

- 4 sea bass fillets, boneless
- 2 tablespoons avocado oil
- 4 scallions, chopped
- ½ cup corn
- ½ cup kalamata olives, pitted and cubed
- 1 teaspoon cayenne pepper
- Juice of ½ lemon
- A pinch of sea salt and black pepper
- 1/3 cup basil, chopped

Directions:

1. Heat up a pan with the oil over medium-high heat, add the scallions and sauté for 2 minutes.
2. Add the fish and cook it for 4 minutes on each side.
3. Add the rest of the ingredients, toss, cook for 4 minutes more, divide between plates and serve.

Nutrition info per serving: calories 270, fat 6, fiber 4, carbs 13, protein 15

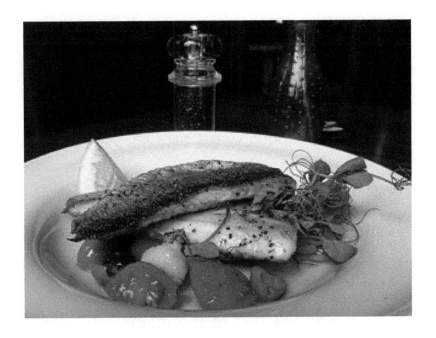

Salmon with Leeks

Prep time: 10 minutes I **Cooking time:** 20 minutes I
Servings: 4

Ingredients:

- 4 salmon fillets, boneless
- 2 tablespoons olive oil
- 2 leeks, sliced
- 1 teaspoon cumin, ground
- ½ teaspoon rosemary, dried
- 1 tablespoon ginger, grated
- 1 tablespoon cilantro, chopped
- 1 teaspoon sweet paprika

Directions:

1. Heat up a pan with the oil over medium heat, add the leeks and sauté for 5 minutes.
2. Add the fish and cook it for 5 minutes on each side.
3. Add the rest of the ingredients, cook the mix for 5 minutes more, divide between plates and serve.

Nutrition info per serving: calories 278, fat 3, fiber 4, carbs 14, protein 15

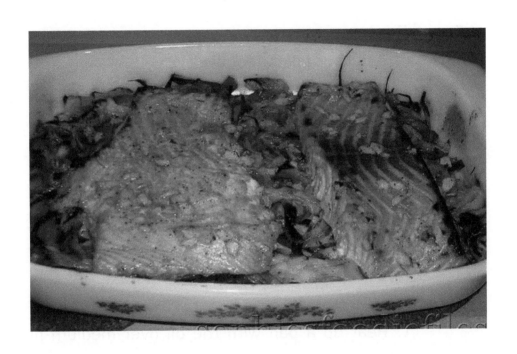

Curry and Coconut Halibut

Prep time: 10 minutes I **Cooking time:** 14 minutes I
Servings: 4

Ingredients:

- 4 halibut fillets, boneless
- 2 tablespoons olive oil
- 4 shallots, chopped
- 1 tablespoon green curry paste
- ¼ cup basil, chopped
- 2 teaspoons coconut aminos
- 1 red chili pepper, chopped
- 1 tablespoon cilantro, chopped

Directions:

1. Heat up a pan with the oil over medium-high heat, add the shallots, curry paste and chili pepper and sauté for 4 minutes.
2. Add the fish and the other ingredients, cook it for 5 minutes on each side, divide between plates and serve.

Nutrition info per serving: calories 210, fat 3, fiber 2, carbs 12, protein 16

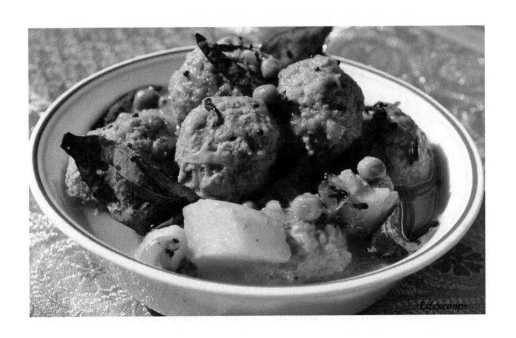

43

Salmon and Rosemary Sweet Potatoes

Prep time: 10 minutes I **Cooking time:** 25 minutes I
Servings: 4

Ingredients:

- 4 salmon fillets, boneless
- 1 garlic cloves, minced
- 2 tablespoons olive oil
- A pinch of salt and black pepper
- 1 yellow onion, sliced
- 2 sweet potatoes, peeled and cut into wedges
- 1 tablespoon rosemary, chopped
- 1 tablespoon lime juice

Directions:

1. Grease a baking dish with the oil, arrange the salmon, garlic, onion and the other ingredients into the dish and bake everything at 380 degrees F for 25 minutes.
2. Divide the mix between plates and serve.

Nutrition info per serving: calories 260, fat 4, fiber 6, carbs 10, protein 16

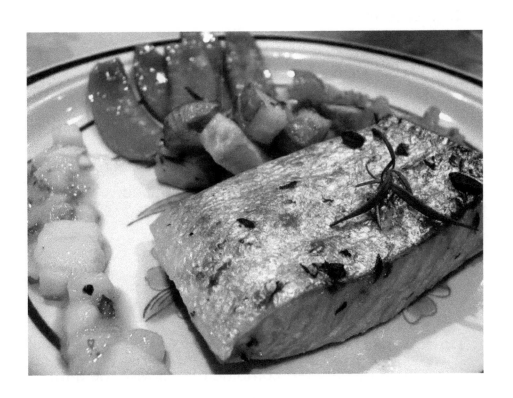

Salmon with Herbs

Prep time: 5 minutes I **Cooking time:** 20 minutes I
Servings: 4

Ingredients:

- 3 tablespoons olive oil
- 4 salmon fillets, boneless
- 4 garlic cloves, minced
- ¼ cup coconut cream
- 1 tablespoon parsley, chopped
- 1 tablespoon rosemary, chopped
- 1 tablespoon basil, chopped
- 1 tablespoon oregano, chopped
- 1 tablespoon pine nuts, toasted
- A pinch of salt and black pepper

Directions:

1. In a blender, combine the oil with the garlic and the other ingredients except the fish and pulse well.
2. Arrange the fish in a roasting pan, add the herbed sauce on top and cook at 380 degrees F for 20 minutes.

3. Divide the mix between plates and serve.

Nutrition info per serving: calories 386, fat 26.8, fiber 1.4, carbs 3.5, protein 35.6

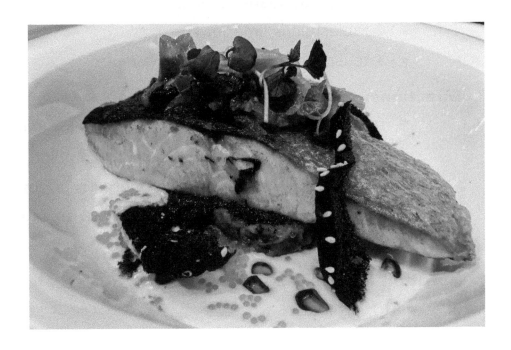

Shrimp and Pinto Beans

Prep time: 5 minutes I **Cooking time:** 12 minutes I

Servings: 4

Ingredients:

- 1 pound shrimp, peeled and deveined
- 2 tablespoons olive oil
- 1 teaspoon cumin, ground
- 4 green onions, chopped
- 1 cup pinto beans, cooked
- 2 tablespoons lime juice
- 1 teaspoon turmeric powder

Directions:

1. Heat up a pan with the oil over medium heat, add the green onions and sauté for 2 minutes.
2. Add the shrimp and the other ingredients, toss, cook over medium heat for another 10 minutes, divide between plates and serve.

Nutrition info per serving: calories 251, fat 12, fiber 2, carbs 13, protein 16

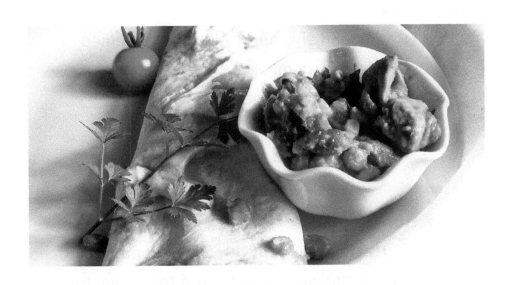

Shrimp with Baby Spinach

Prep time: 10 minutes I **Cooking time:** 10 minutes I
Servings: 4

Ingredients:

- 1 pound shrimp, peeled and deveined
- 2 tablespoons olive oil
- 1 tablespoon lime juice
- 1 cup baby spinach
- A pinch of sea salt and black pepper
- 1 tablespoon chives, chopped

Directions:

1. Heat up the pan with the oil over medium heat, add the shrimp and sauté for 5 minutes.
2. Add the spinach and the remaining ingredients, toss, cook the mix for another 5 minutes, divide between plates and serve.

Nutrition info per serving: calories 206, fat 6, fiber 4, carbs 7, protein 17

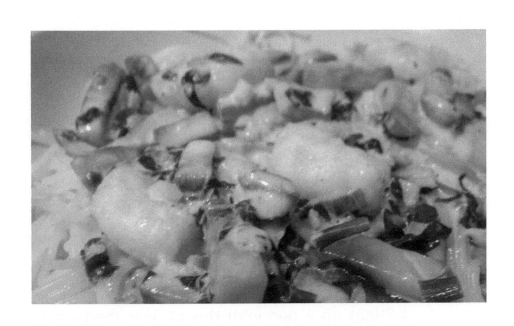

Cod and Peppers

Prep time: 10 minutes I **Cooking time:** 15 minutes I
Servings: 4

Ingredients:

- 4 cod fillets, boneless
- 2 tablespoons olive oil
- 4 spring onions, chopped
- Juice of 1 lime
- 1 red bell pepper, cut into strips
- 1 green bell pepper, cut into strips
- 2 teaspoons parsley, chopped
- A pinch of salt and black pepper

Directions:

1. Heat up a pan with the oil over medium heat, add the bell peppers and the onions and sauté for 5 minutes.
2. Add the fish and the rest of the ingredients, cook the mix for 10 minutes more, flipping the fish halfway.
3. Divide the mix between plates and serve.

Nutrition info per serving: calories 180, fat 5, fiber 1, carbs 7, protein 11

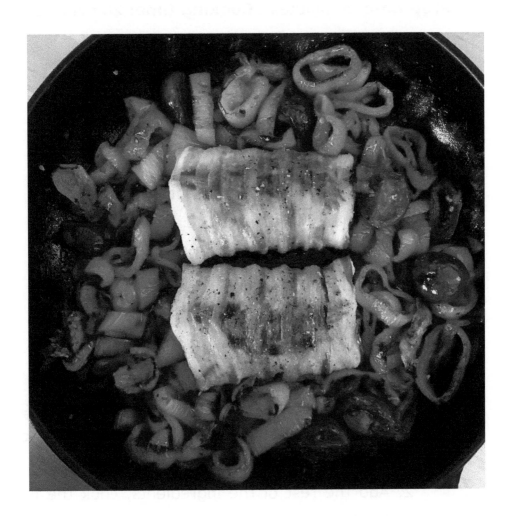

Cod with Avocado and Peppers Pan

Prep time: 5 minutes I **Cooking time:** 20 minutes I
Servings: 4

Ingredients:

- 1 pound cod fillets, boneless and cubed
- 2 tablespoons avocado oil
- 1 avocado, peeled, pitted and cubed
- 1 red sweet pepper, cut into strips
- 1 tablespoon lemon juice
- ¼ cup parsley, chopped
- 1 tablespoon tomato paste
- ½ cup veggie stock
- A pinch of sea salt and black pepper

Directions:

1. Heat up a pan with the oil over medium-high heat, add the fish and cook for 3 minutes on each side.
2. Add the rest of the ingredients, cook the mix for 14 minutes more over medium heat, divide between plates and serve.

Nutrition info per serving: calories 160, fat 2, fiber 2, carbs 4, protein 7

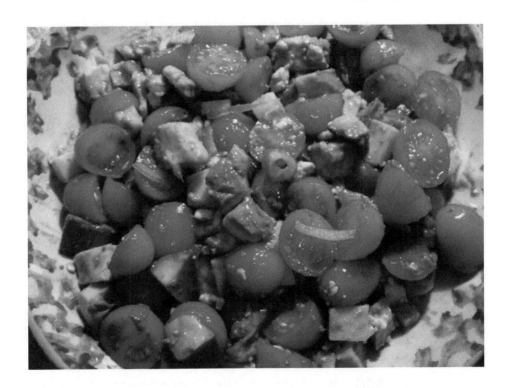

Shrimp and Zucchinis

Prep time: 5 minutes I **Cooking time:** 8 minutes I
Servings: 4

Ingredients:

- 1 pound shrimp, peeled and deveined
- 2 tablespoons avocado oil
- 2 zucchinis, sliced
- Juice of 1 lime
- A pinch of salt and black pepper
- 2 red chilies, chopped
- 3 garlic cloves, minced
- 1 tablespoon balsamic vinegar

Directions:

1. Heat up a pan with the oil over medium-high heat, add the shrimp, garlic and the chilies and cook for 3 minutes.
2. Add the rest of the ingredients, toss, cook everything for 5 minutes more, divide between plates and serve.

Nutrition info per serving: calories 211, fat 5, fiber 2, carbs 11, protein 15

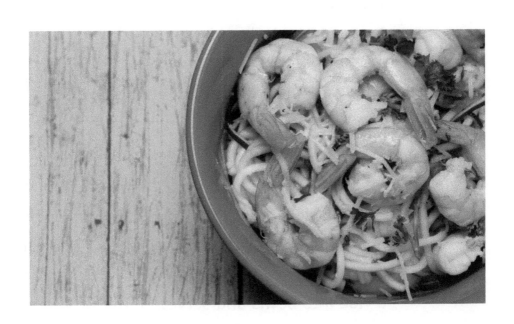

Lemon Rosemary Scallops

Prep time: 10 minutes I **Cooking time:** 10 minutes I
Servings: 4

Ingredients:

- 2 tablespoons olive oil
- 1 pound sea scallops
- ½ teaspoon rosemary, dried
- ½ cup veggie stock
- 2 garlic cloves, minced
- Juice of ½ lemon

Directions:

1. Heat up a pan with the oil over medium-high heat, add the garlic, the scallops and the other ingredients, cook everything for 10 minutes, divide into bowls and serve.

Nutrition info per serving: calories 170, fat 5, fiber 2, carbs 8, protein 10

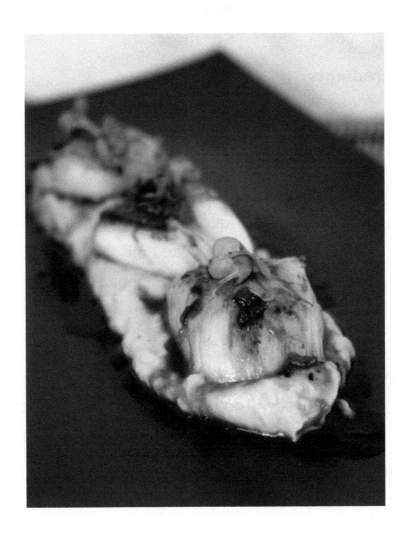

Crab and Kale Salad

Prep time: 5 minutes I **Cooking time:** 0 minutes I
Servings: 4

Ingredients:

- 1 cup crab meat, cooked
- 1 pound shrimp, peeled, deveined and cooked
- 1 cup cherry tomatoes, halved
- 1 cucumber, sliced
- 2 cups baby kale
- 2 tablespoons avocado oil
- 1 tablespoon chives, chopped
- 1 tablespoon lemon juice
- A pinch of salt and black pepper

Directions:

1. In a bowl, combine the shrimp with the crab meat and the other ingredients, toss and serve.

Nutrition info per serving: calories 203, fat 12, fiber 6, carbs 12, protein 9

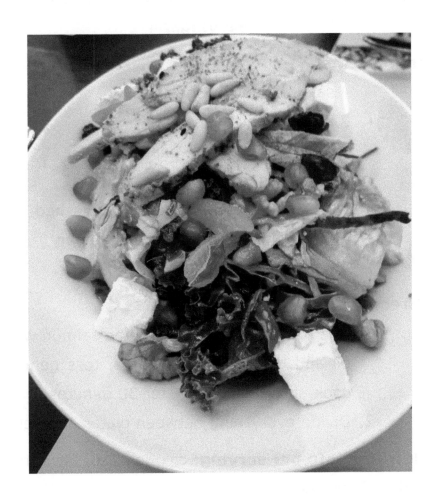

Salmon with Paprika Tomatoes

Prep time: 10 minutes I **Cooking time:** 30 minutes I
Servings: 4

Ingredients:

- 4 salmon fillets, boneless
- 2 tablespoons avocado oil
- 2 tablespoons sweet paprika
- 2 tomatoes, cut into wedges
- ¼ teaspoon red pepper flakes, crushed
- A pinch of sea salt and black pepper
- 4 garlic cloves, minced

Directions:

1. In a roasting pan, combine the salmon with the oil and the other ingredients, toss gently and cook at 370 degrees F for 30 minutes.
2. Divide everything between plates and serve.

Nutrition info per serving: calories 210, fat 2, fiber 4, carbs 13, protein 10

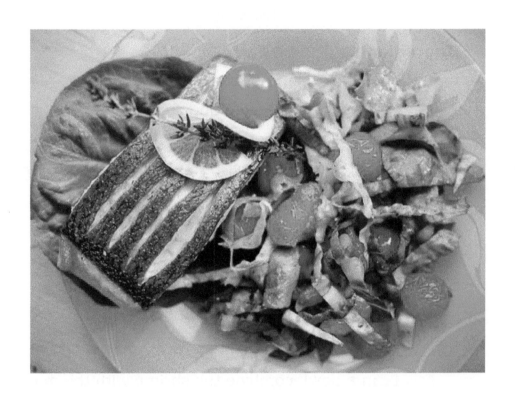

Shrimp and Mango Salad

Prep time: 5 minutes I **Cooking time:** 0 minutes I
Servings: 4

Ingredients:

- 1 pound shrimp, cooked, peeled and deveined
- 2 mangoes, peeled and cubed
- 3 scallions, chopped
- 1 cup baby spinach
- 1 cup baby arugula
- 1 jalapeno, chopped
- 2 tablespoons olive oil
- 1 tablespoon lime juice
- A pinch of salt and black pepper

Directions:

1. In a bowl, combine the shrimp with the mango, scallions and the other ingredients, toss and serve.

Nutrition info per serving: calories 210, fat 2, fiber 3, carbs 13, protein 8

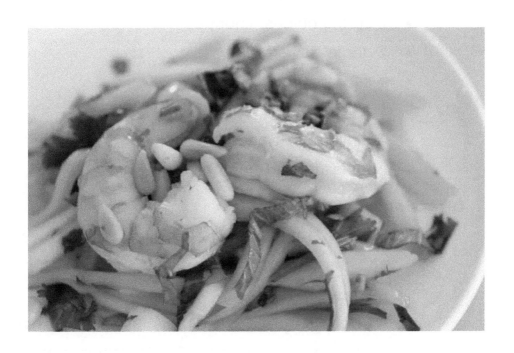

Creamy Cod

Prep time: 5 minutes I **Cooking time:** 20 minutes I
Servings: 4

Ingredients:

- 2 tablespoons olive oil
- 1 pound cod fillets, boneless and cubed
- 2 spring onions, chopped
- 2 garlic cloves, minced
- 1 cup coconut cream
- ¼ cup chives, chopped
- A pinch of salt and black pepper
- 2 tablespoons Dijon mustard

Directions:

1. Heat up a pan with the oil over medium heat, add the garlic and the onions and sauté for 5 minutes.
2. Add the fish and the other ingredients, toss, cook over medium heat for 15 minutes more, divide into bowls and serve.

Nutrition info per serving: calories 211, fat 5, fiber 5, carbs 6, protein 15

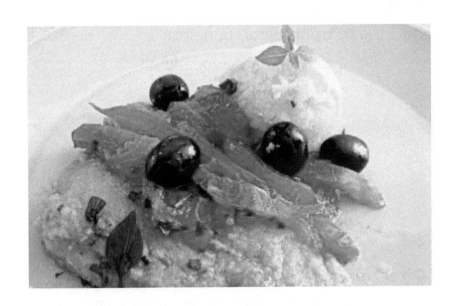

Trout and Walnuts Cilantro Sauce

Prep time: 5 minutes I **Cooking time:** 15 minutes I
Servings: 4

Ingredients:

- 4 trout fillets, boneless
- 2 tablespoons avocado oil
- 1 cup cilantro, chopped
- 2 tablespoons lemon juice
- ½ cup coconut cream
- 1 tablespoon walnuts, chopped
- A pinch of salt and black pepper
- 3 teaspoons lemon zest, grated

Directions:

1. In a blender, combine the cilantro with the cream and the other ingredients except the fish and the oil and pulse well.
2. Heat up a pan with the oil over medium heat, add the fish and cook for 4 minutes on each side.
3. Add the cilantro sauce, toss gently and cook over medium heat for 7 minutes more.
4. Divide the mix between plates and serve.

Nutrition info per serving: calories 212, fat 14.6, fiber 1.3, carbs 2.9, protein 18

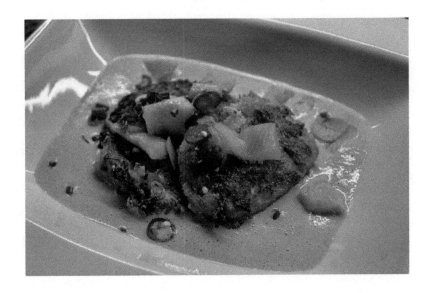

Cilantro Tilapia

Prep time: 5 minutes I **Cooking time:** 12 minutes I
Servings: 4

Ingredients:

- 4 tilapia fillets, boneless
- 2 tablespoons olive oil
- 2 tablespoons lemon juice
- 1 teaspoon basil, dried
- 1 tablespoon cilantro, chopped

Directions:

1. Heat up a pan with the oil over medium heat, add the fish and cook for 5 minutes on each side.
2. Add the rest of the ingredients, toss gently, cook for 2 minutes more, divide between plates and serve.

Nutrition info per serving: calories 201, fat 8.6, fiber 0, carbs 0.2, protein 31.6

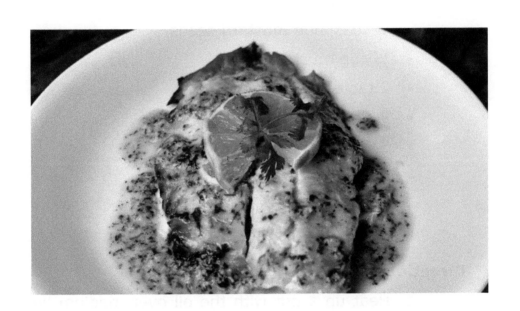

Salmon and Green Chilies Mix

Prep time: 5 minutes I **Cooking time:** 14 minutes I
Servings: 4

Ingredients:

- 4 salmon fillets, boneless
- ½ teaspoon mustard seeds
- ½ cup mustard
- 2 tablespoons olive oil
- 4 scallions, chopped
- Salt and black pepper to the taste
- 2 green chilies, chopped
- ¼ teaspoon cumin, ground
- ¼ cup parsley, chopped

Directions:

1. Heat up a pot with the oil over medium heat, add the scallions and the chilies and cook for 2 minutes.
2. Add the fish and cook for 4 minutes on each side.

3. Add the remaining ingredients, toss, cook everything for 4 more minutes, divide between plates and serve.

Nutrition info per serving: calories 397, fat 23.9, fiber 3.5, carbs 8,5, protein 40

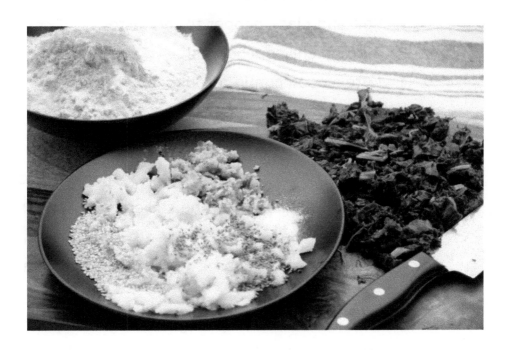

Salmon and Green Chilies Mix

Prep time: 5 minutes I **Cooking time:** 14 minutes I
Servings: 4

Ingredients:

- 4 salmon fillets, boneless
- ½ teaspoon mustard seeds
- ½ cup mustard
- 2 tablespoons olive oil
- 4 scallions, chopped
- Salt and black pepper to the taste
- 2 green chilies, chopped
- ¼ teaspoon cumin, ground
- ¼ cup parsley, chopped

Directions:

3. Heat up a pot with the oil over medium heat, add the scallions and the chilies and cook for 2 minutes.
4. Add the fish and cook for 4 minutes on each side.
5. Add the remaining ingredients, toss, cook everything for 4 more minutes, divide between plates and serve.

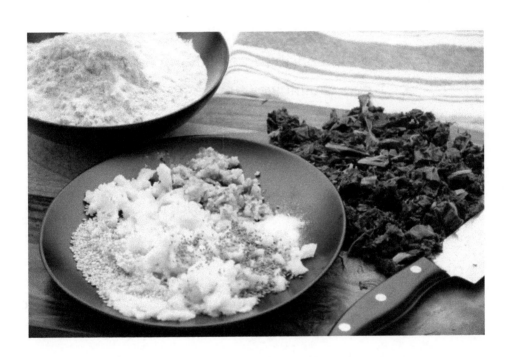

Shrimp and Turmeric Cauliflower Mix

Prep time: 10 minutes I **Cooking time:** 10 minutes I
Servings: 4

Ingredients:

- 2 tablespoons olive oil
- 1 pound shrimp, peeled and deveined
- 1 cup cauliflower florets
- 2 tablespoons lemon juice
- 2 tablespoons garlic, minced
- 1 teaspoon cumin, ground
- 1 teaspoon turmeric powder
- Salt and black pepper to the taste

Directions:

1. Heat up a pan with the oil over medium-high heat, add the garlic and sauté for 2 minutes.
2. Add the shrimp and cook for 4 minutes more.
3. Add the remaining ingredients, toss, cook the mix for 4 minutes, divide between plates and serve

Nutrition info per serving: calories 200, fat 5.3, fiber 3, carbs 11, protein 6

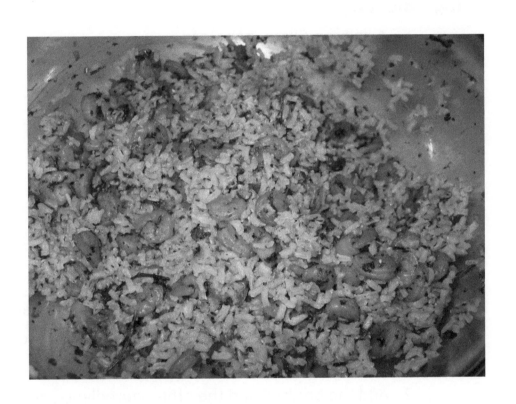

Tuna with Broccoli

Prep time: 5 minutes I **Cooking time:** 15 minutes I
Servings: 4

Ingredients:

- 4 salmon fillets, boneless
- 1 teaspoon coriander, ground
- 1 cup broccoli florets
- 2 tablespoons lemon juice
- 2 tablespoons avocado oil
- 1 tablespoon lemon zest, grated
- A pinch of salt and black pepper
- 2 tablespoons cilantro, chopped

Directions:

1. Heat up a pan with the oil over medium heat, add the fish and cook for 4 minutes on each side.
2. Add the broccoli and the other ingredients, cook the mix for 7 more minutes, divide between plates and serve.

Nutrition info per serving: calories 210, fat 4.7, fiber 2, carbs 11, protein 17

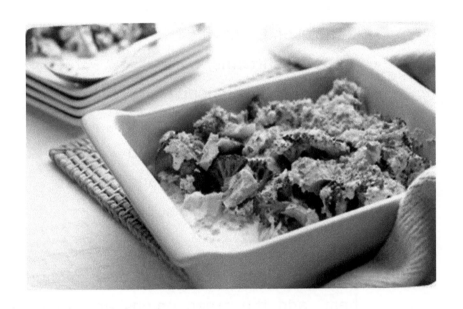

Flounder with Mushrooms

Prep time: 10 minutes I **Cooking time:** 20 minutes I
Servings: 4

Ingredients:

- 4 flounder fillets, boneless
- 2 tablespoons olive oil
- 1 cup mushrooms, sliced
- 3 green onions, chopped
- 1 tablespoon lime juice
- ¼ teaspoon nutmeg, ground
- ¼ cup almonds, toasted and chopped
- A pinch of salt and black pepper

Directions:

1. Heat up a pan with the oil over medium-high heat, add the green onions and sauté for 5 minutes.
2. Add the mushrooms and cook for 5 minutes more.
3. Add the fish and the other ingredients, cook it for 5 minutes on each side, divide between plates and serve.

Nutrition info per serving: calories 250, fat 10, fiber 3.3, carbs 7, protein 20

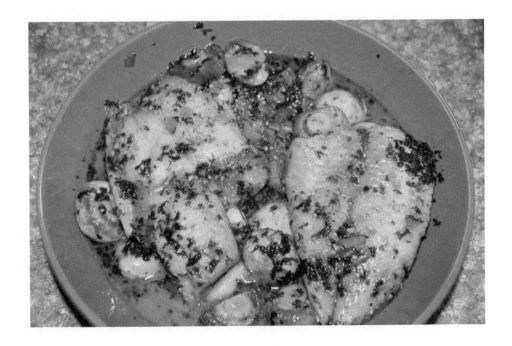

Spicy Shrimp with Rice

Prep time: 10 minutes I **Cooking time:** 25 minutes I
Servings: 4

Ingredients:

- 1 pound shrimp, peeled and deveined
- 1 cup black rice
- 2 cups chicken stock
- 4 scallions, chopped
- 1 teaspoon chili powder
- 1 teaspoon sweet paprika
- 2 tablespoons avocado oil
- A pinch of salt and black pepper

Directions:

1. Heat up a pan with the oil over medium-high heat, add the scallions and sauté for 5 minutes.
2. Add the rice and the other ingredients except the shrimp, and cook the mix for 15 minutes.
3. Add the shrimp, cook everything for another 5 minutes, divide into bowls and serve.

Nutrition info per serving: calories 240, fat 7, fiber 6, carbs 8, protein 14

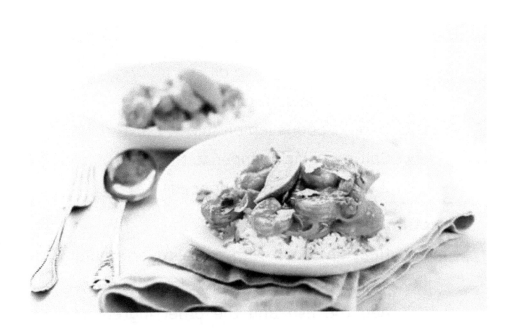

Dill Sea Bass

Prep time: 5 minutes I **Cooking time:** 12 minutes I
Servings: 4

Ingredients:

- 4 sea bass fillets, boneless
- 2 tablespoons olive oil
- 3 spring onions, chopped
- 2 tablespoons lemon juice
- Salt and black pepper to the taste
- 2 tablespoons dill, chopped

Directions:

1. Heat up a pan with the oil over medium heat, add the onions and sauté for 2 minutes.
2. Add the fish and the other ingredients, cook everything for 5 minutes on each side, divide the mix between plates and serve.

Nutrition info per serving: calories 214, fat 12, fiber 4, carbs 7, protein 17

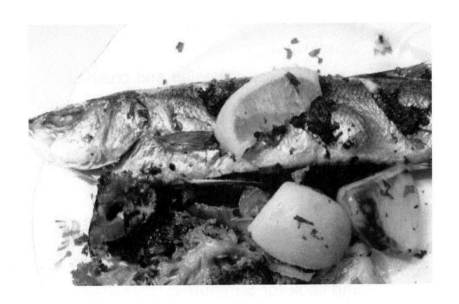

Trout with Coconut Tomato Sauce

Prep time: 4 minutes I **Cooking time:** 15 minutes I
Servings: 4

Ingredients:

- 4 trout fillets, boneless
- 2 spring onions, chopped
- 2 tablespoons olive oil
- 1 cup tomatoes, peeled and crushed
- ¼ cup coconut cream
- 1 tablespoon chives, chopped
- A pinch of salt and black pepper

Directions:

1. Heat up a pan with the oil over medium heat, add the spring onions, tomatoes and the cream and cook for 5 minutes.
2. Add the fish and the rest of the ingredients, toss, cook everything for 10 minutes more, divide between plates and serve.

Nutrition info per serving: calories 200, fat 5, fiber 6, carbs 12, protein 12

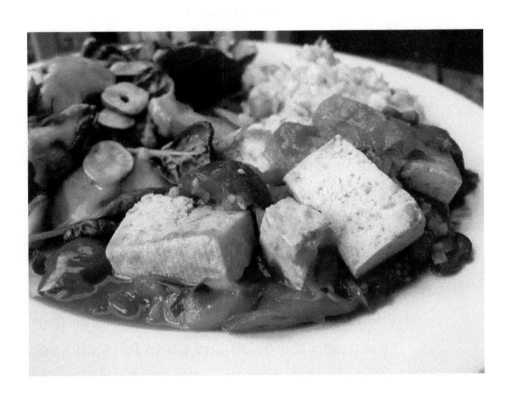

Salmon and Cilantro Roasted Peppers

Prep time: 5 minutes I **Cooking time:** 25 minutes I
Servings: 4

Ingredients:

- 1 cup roasted red peppers, cut into strips
- 4 salmon fillets, boneless
- ¼ cup chicken stock
- 2 tablespoons olive oil
- 1 yellow onion, chopped
- 1 tablespoon cilantro, chopped
- A pinch of sea salt and black pepper

Directions:

1. Heat up a pan with the oil over medium-high heat, add the onion and sauté for 5 minutes.
2. Add the fish and cook for 5 minutes on each side.
3. Add the rest of the ingredients, introduce the pan in the oven and cook at 390 degrees F for 10 minutes.
4. Divide the mix between plates and serve.

Nutrition info per serving: calories 265, fat 7, fiber 5, carbs 15, protein 16

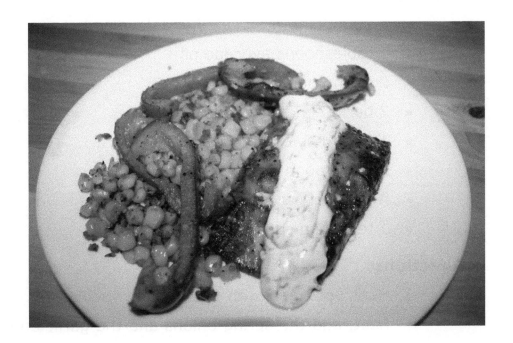

Lemon and Garlic Shrimp and Beets

Prep time: 10 minutes I **Cooking time:** 10 minutes I
Servings: 4

Ingredients:

- 1 pound shrimp, peeled and deveined
- 2 tablespoons avocado oil
- 2 spring onions, chopped
- 2 garlic cloves, minced
- 1 beet, peeled and cubed
- 1 tablespoon lemon juice
- A pinch of sea salt and black pepper
- 1 teaspoon coconut aminos

Directions:

1. Heat up a pan with the oil over medium-high heat, add the spring onions and the garlic and sauté for 2 minutes.
2. Add the shrimp and the other ingredients, toss, cook the mix for 8 minutes, divide into bowls and serve.

Nutrition info per serving: calories 281, fat 6, fiber 7, carbs 11, protein 8

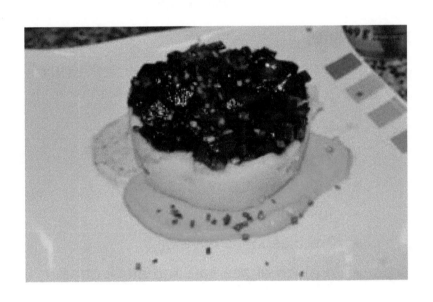

Parsley and Lime Shrimp

Prep time: 5 minutes I **Cooking time:** 10 minutes I
Servings: 4

Ingredients:

- 1 pound shrimp, peeled and deveined
- 2 garlic cloves, minced
- 1 cup corn
- ½ cup veggie stock
- 1 bunch parsley, chopped
- Juice of 1 lime
- 2 tablespoons olive oil
- A pinch of sea salt and black pepper

Directions:

1. Heat up a pan with the oil over medium-high heat, add the garlic and the corn and sauté for 2 minutes.
2. Add the shrimp and the other ingredients, toss, cook everything for 8 minutes more, divide between plates and serve.

Nutrition info per serving: calories 345, fat 11.2, fiber 4.5, carbs 15, protein 5.6

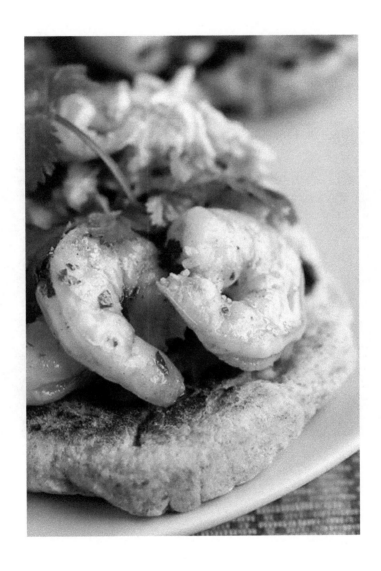

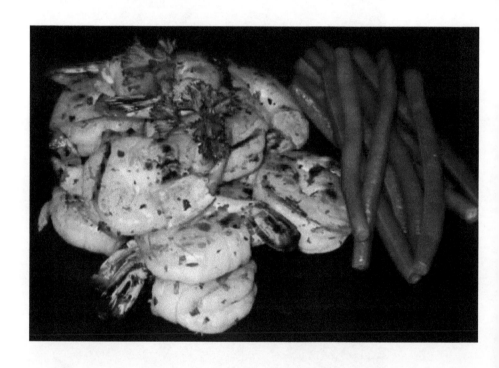

Cumin Shrimp and Almonds

Prep time: 10 minutes I **Cooking time:** 10 minutes I
Servings: 4

Ingredients:

- 1 pound shrimp, peeled and deveined
- 2 tablespoons chili paste
- A pinch of sea salt and black pepper
- 1 tablespoon olive oil
- 1 cup pineapple, peeled and cubed
- ½ teaspoon ginger, grated
- 2 teaspoons almonds, chopped
- 2 tablespoons cilantro, chopped

Directions:

1. Heat up a pan with the oil over medium-high heat, add the ginger and the chili paste, stir and cook for 2 minutes.
2. Add the shrimp and the other ingredients, toss, cook the mix for 8 minutes more, divide into bowls and serve.

Nutrition info per serving: calories 261, fat 4, fiber 7, carbs 15, protein 8

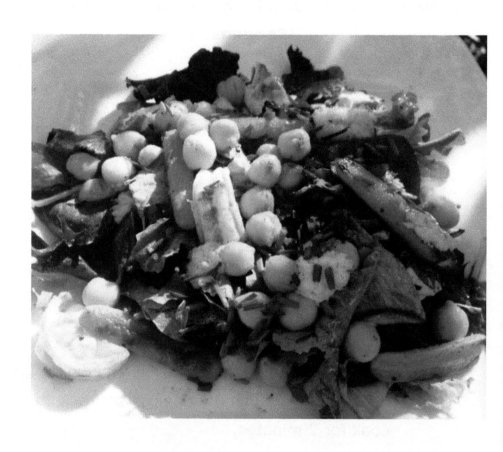

Tilapia and Red Beans

Prep time: 5 minutes I **Cooking time:** 20 minutes I
Servings: 4

Ingredients:

- 1 tablespoon olive oil
- 2 tablespoons green curry paste
- 4 tilapia fillets, boneless
- Juice of ½ lime
- 1 cup red kidney beans, cooked
- 1 tablespoon parsley, chopped

Directions:

1. Heat up a pan with the oil over medium heat, add the fish and cook for 5 minutes on each side.
2. Add the rest of the ingredients, toss gently, cook over medium heat for 10 minutes more, divide between plates and serve.

Nutrition info per serving: calories 271, fat 4, fiber 6, carbs 14, protein 7

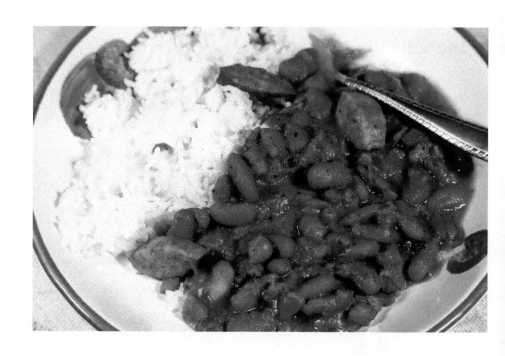

Shrimp with Corn and Olives

Prep time: 5 minutes I **Cooking time:** 10 minutes I
Servings: 4

Ingredients:

- 2 tablespoons olive oil
- 1 pound shrimp, peeled and deveined
- 1 teaspoon rosemary, dried
- 1 cup corn
- 1 cup black olives, pitted and halved
- 1 teaspoon smoked paprika
- A pinch of sea salt and black pepper

Directions:

1. Heat up a pan with the oil over medium-high heat, add the shrimp, rosemary and the other ingredients, toss, cook for 10 minutes, divide into bowls and serve.

Nutrition info per serving: calories 271, fat 4, fiber 6, carbs 14, protein 15

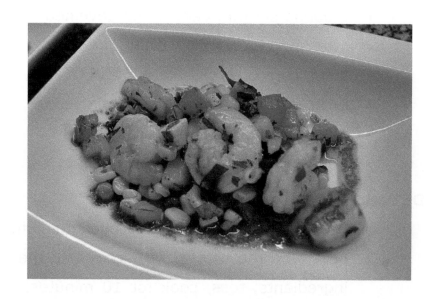

Citrus Scallops

Prep time: 5 minutes I **Cooking time:** 10 minutes I
Servings: 4

Ingredients:

- 1 pound sea scallops
- 4 scallions, chopped
- 2 tablespoons olive oil
- 1 tablespoon orange juice
- 1 tablespoon cilantro, chopped
- A pinch of salt and black pepper

Directions:

1. Heat up a pan with the oil over medium-high heat, add the scallops, the scallions and the other ingredients, toss, cook for 10 minutes, divide into bowls and serve.

Nutrition info per serving: calories 300, fat 4, fiber 4, carbs 14, protein 17

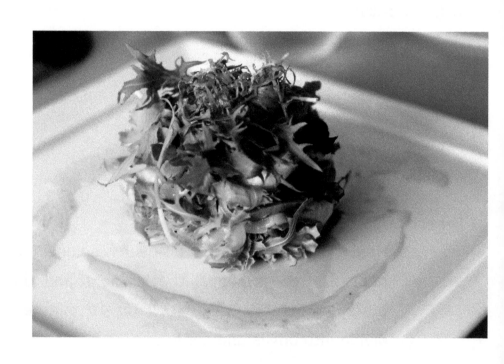

Shrimp with Leeks and Carrots

Prep time: 5 minutes I **Cooking time:** 10 minutes I

Servings: 4

Ingredients:

- 1 pound shrimp, peeled and deveined
- 1 cup leeks, sliced
- 2 tablespoons olive oil
- ¼ cup vegetable stock
- 2 tablespoons rosemary, chopped
- 2 cups baby carrots, peeled
- 1 tablespoon lime juice
- A pinch of sea salt and black pepper

Directions:

1. Heat up a pan with the oil over medium-high heat, add the carrots, rosemary and the other ingredients except the shrimp, toss and cook for 5 minutes.
2. Add the shrimp, cook the mix for 5 minutes more, divide into bowls and serve.

Nutrition info per serving: calories 271, fat 6, fiber 7, carbs 14, protein 18

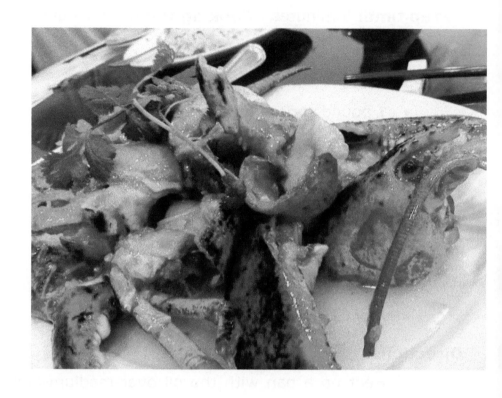

Cod and Barley

Prep time: 10 minutes I **Cooking time:** 25 minutes I
Servings: 4

Ingredients:

- 3 scallions, chopped
- 2 cups chicken stock
- 1 pound cod fillets, boneless and cubed
- 1 cup barley
- 2 tablespoons olive oil
- 2 celery stalks, chopped
- A pinch of salt and black pepper
- 1 tablespoon coriander, chopped

Directions:

1. Heat up a pan with the oil over medium-high heat, add the scallions and the celery and sauté for 5 minutes.
2. Add the fish and cook for 5 minutes more.
3. Add the rest of the ingredients, toss, cook over medium heat for 15 minutes more, divide everything between plates and serve.

Nutrition info per serving: calories 261, fat 4, fiber 6, carbs 14, protein 7

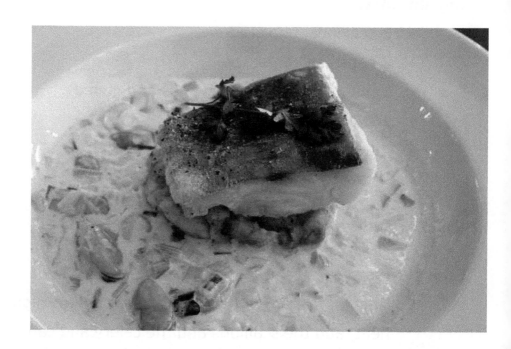

Shrimp and Balsamic Sweet Peppers

Prep time: 5 minutes I **Cooking time:** 12 minutes I
Servings: 4

Ingredients:

- 1 pound shrimp, peeled and deveined
- 2 tablespoons avocado oil
- 2 spring onions, chopped
- 2 sweet peppers, cut into strips
- 1 tablespoon balsamic vinegar
- 1 tablespoon chives, minced
- A pinch of sea salt and black pepper

Directions:

1. Heat up a pan with the oil over medium-high heat, add the spring onions, peppers and chives, stir and cook for 4 minutes.
2. Add the shrimp and the rest of the ingredients, toss, cook over medium heat for 8 minutes more, divide into bowls and serve.

Nutrition info per serving: calories 191, fat 3.3, fiber 8,5 carbs 11.3, protein 29.3

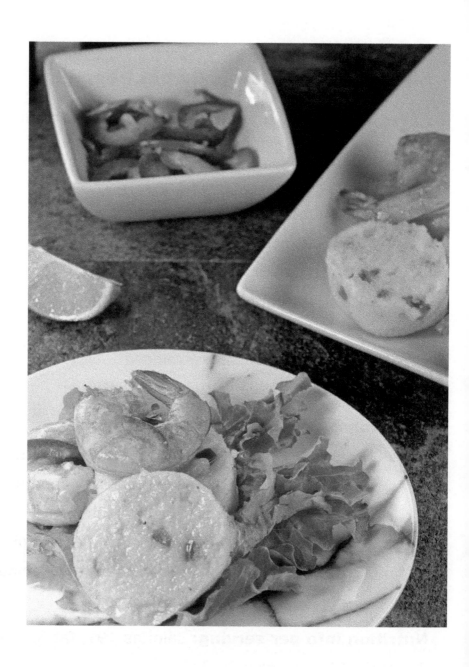

Cumin Snapper Mix

Prep time: 5 minutes I **Cooking time:** 20 minutes I
Servings: 4

Ingredients:

- 2 tablespoons olive oil
- 2 garlic cloves, minced
- 4 snapper fillets, boneless, skinless and cubed
- 1 tomato, cubed
- 1 zucchini, cubed
- 1 tablespoon coriander, chopped
- ½ teaspoon cumin, ground
- ½ teaspoon rosemary, dried
- A pinch of salt and black pepper

Directions:

1. Heat up a pan with the oil over medium-high heat, add the garlic, tomato and zucchini and cook for 5 minutes.
2. Add the fish and the other ingredients, toss, cook the mix for 15 minutes more, divide it into bowls and serve.

Nutrition info per serving: calories 251, fat 4, fiber 6, carbs 14, protein 7

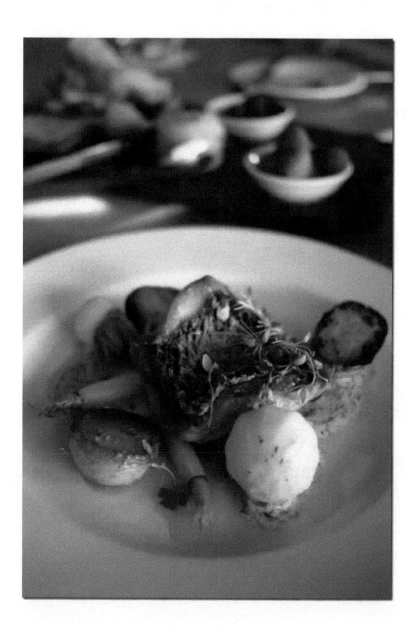